Eyelash Pulling

How to Cure Eyelash and Eyebrow Trichotillomania

2nd Edition

By Amy Foxwell

Table of Contents

Welcome to the Trich Stop System

Sharing My Story

A Word About the Trich Stop System

Background

 Why do I Pull Out my Eyelashes and Eyebrows?

 What is Hair Pulling Disorder or Trichotillomania?

 What Causes Trichotillomania?

 Who Suffers from Trichotillomania?

 The Phases of Trichotillomania

Treatment

 Cognitive Behavior Theory

 Medication

Amino Acids

Therapy

Living With Hair Pulling

Embracing Your Unique You

Being an 'Ex' Eyelash Puller

Setbacks and How to Deal with Them

Hair Pulling Tools

The Success Mindset: Using Visualization

Auto-hypnosis

Coming Around the Problem

8 Step Trich Stop System

Trich Stop Tips

Dealing with Others

Facts About Hair

Recommended Resources

Using the Trich Stop Worksheet and Journal

My Trich Stop Success Journal

A Special Offer

The Trich Stop Loved One's Guide

Welcome to the Trich Stop System

Thank you for purchasing the Trich Stop Kit and congratulations. You have taken the first step to a new you. I am delighted to share this method that helped me to stop pulling my eyelashes and eyebrows out and is sure to give you long-lasting results. I have spent much time researching and developing this book for it to be as effective as possible. This is the second edition of this book, with additional sections, additional tips, recommended reading, and a special 'Loved Ones' section that you can use either to help a friend or family member, or to communicate to others about your own condition. In any case, to see lasting results follow the instructions and most of all, be kind to yourself as you embark on this journey.

My best,

Sharing My Story

Over the years I have been in contact with many people – both ex- hair pullers and skin pickers, as well as those who are still working through their conditions. In these exchanges I realize that exchanging stories is an important step in healing. We can take both solace and encouragement in knowing that we are not alone, that it is indeed possible to stop our obsessive compulsive behaviors, and that others have done so. Therefore I would like to share my own story with you. I hope that by sharing this with you it can help you in your own treatment.

I suffered from both hair pulling and skin picking as early as I can remember. I have a vivid memory as a child saving all of my eyelashes in a metal box, totally oblivious to how strange this was until people started wondering why I had no eyelashes. Looking back I have no idea if this was related to a stressful childhood, or just that I was predisposed to this condition, but in any case I continued to pull out my eyelashes and eyebrows, sometimes more and sometimes less.

As I hit my twenties the condition got much worse. While modern society idolizes being young, many young adults find it a difficult time in their lives, as did I. However I was still unaware that I had a veritable problem and continued to pull out my eyelashes and eyebrows, spending time to conceal the patches by searching high and low for an eye pencil to fill in my brows and lashes and other disguises. I was so envious of the other members of my family who had lovely, long lashes that seemed to mock my own bald patches and made things even more frustrating for me. If I could only stop, just LOOK at the lashes I'd have.

Emotionally, living with my eyelash pulling and other obsessive-compulsive behaviors was a constant heaviness in my life. It weighed down on me, always there, in the back of my mind, whether I was fighting with the urges, making sure my eyebrows were filled in, dealing with the frustration or puzzling over what was wrong with me. I was living a continuous battle with myself. Every morning and every evening I would give myself a pep talk, telling myself that I would quit, I would "just stop" (yes, unbelievable, I said those very words to myself, over and over again, those words that others say to hair pullers and that are so terribly frustrating to hear), believing that merely having some self-control would put an end to my actions, that surely I was an intelligent person and I could do such a simple thing. I would convince myself in the morning that 'THIS DAY WOULD BE MY LAST DAY I PULLED MY EYELASHES OUT' only to then be faced with myself and bald patches that evening, having failed YET AGAIN. The mixture of frustration and damage to my self-confidence was deeply rooted and misunderstood, even by myself.

Despite the lack of eyelashes or eyebrows, I continued with my hair pulling which was really very much out of control. However crazy as it sounds though, amazingly I didn't even realize that I had an obsessive-compulsive 'condition'. But one fine day, much later in life, I mentioned in passing to my doctor that I had a place that was continually itchy and where I was 'losing' my eyelashes (I was too embarrassed to admit that I was pulling them out, even to my doctor who I was asking for help). She took one look at me declared that I was suffering from a condition known as 'Trichotillomania' (what is THAT? Even the name of the condition is strange) and I should consider starting therapy.

That was both a terrible day ("I have a 'CONDITION'? I don't want a 'condition'") and a wonderful day ("So, I'm not crazy.

There is a legitimate reason to this. And if this is truly a condition, then I can then find a 'treatment' that works.").

I immediately went home and started to do some research. Putting a name to what was happening to me and identifying the condition was the beginning of a huge change for me. Once I started reading up on my condition, while I felt ashamed, I actually felt a sort of freedom. I experienced all sorts of emotions, from denial ("I am a 'normal' successful person, I can't suffer from obsessive compulsive disorder!") to shame ('there is something wrong with me') to relief ('there are others out there just like me! And there is a reason I do this. I'm NOT crazy, and I'm NOT alone). In any case, at least there was a reason behind my actions. That was a turning point for me. I think that awareness and true understanding is absolutely essential for eyelash pullers to advance.

Armed with this information and encouragement, and loath to get outside help, I began a process of gathering research and ideas for helping me through my condition. Initially for my own treatment, I tried many different methods and put together a system that gave me a reassuring structure to work within. After trying products such as Nioxin and Latisse, I also searched high and low for an all-natural product to use in my treatment (having used essential oils and homeopathic treatments with much success throughout my life). Not finding anything, I created my own all-natural oil using olive oil and plant essences from my own garden as well as those produced organically around me.

And then I began applying all the methods I had found, testing and refining them until I eventually worked through my obsessive-compulsive disorders. During this process I met many people and had many enriching exchanges, until one day I realized that others suffering from these conditions could also benefit from the work that I had done. So I decided to view this experience as a way that I could give to others. That I would not have suffered from this condition in vain. And so I put together the Trich Stop System for hair and eyelash pullers.

I am often asked if I ever have any relapses. The answer is that I still do feel occasional urges and I still have a hotspot that often acts up. However I am now able to control the urge and resist. But that just serves to remind me how much progress I have made and that I am indeed the one in control. Each and every victory makes me stronger.

And so I wish you much success in your own journey with Trichotillomania. While I will go over the following tips in depth in this book, along with others, the list below are the essential things that I found helped me most in my struggle with hair pulling. Note these down (or tear out the copy in the Workbook) and refer to them often as a reminder.

My 7 top tips to keep your eyelash pulling under control:

1. Recognize the condition, read up, do some research, really understand what you are confronting.

2. Believe that it is possible to get your condition under control. Surround yourself with a positive support group and have faith.

3. Get a systematized plan in place. You can't just expect to stop, and surely we all know that 'willpower' is just not the answer. So you need to put a very clear plan in place.

4. Try different methods to see which one works for you. Every person is different, so methods will have differing results depending on the person. Try

visualization, journalizing, and mediation. All of these methods have their merits. The best option in my opinion is to have a mix of methods.

5. Use something (natural) to stroke on the area. For me this was key because it helped me not only relieve the nagging feelings, but more importantly, it helped me rewire my brain and change the pulling action to a stroking action. I still find myself stroking or rubbing when I can feel an urge coming on. That is a heck of a lot better than pulling!

6. Cut out chemicals in your diet (processed foods, sugars, etc) and in your cosmetics. And get as healthy as you can.

7. Finally, be KIND TO YOUR SELF. We all know that getting these conditions under control is very difficult. So if you slip up, then give yourself a break, pick yourself up, dust yourself off and start again. Stopping is a gradual process, so be happy with any

progress you have made and keep at it. Don't get discouraged.

There are many people out there having the same experience of Trichotillomania as you; you are not alone.

A Word about the Trich Stop System

Whether you have been battling with Trichotillomania for many years, or have just begun to see symptoms of this condition, you must personally resolve to take control of the situation. And that is what the Trich Stop System is for; to help you succeed in tackling your own personal Trichotillomania condition. Everyone is different and everyone's condition is different. However there are some underlying causes and remedies that are common to everyone. You will need to understand as much as you can about your condition and then put these action steps in place to help you beat it. The key to know is that this can be done. **YOU CAN STOP PULLING YOUR EYELASHES AND EYEBROWS OUT**. You just need the support and plan in place to help you. And that is where the Trich Stop System comes in. Read this manual and begin the steps, using an all-natural oil such as the Trich Stop Hairgrowth Oil (see the end of this book for more information and a special reader offer or refer to: http://trichotillomaniastop.com/hair-growth-oil/) to help you achieve your goals. You will see immediate improvements. Congratulate yourself and recognize that if you can make these first steps towards improvement, then the final goal of stopping your eyelash pulling is within your reach.

So, now that you know that you will succeed, let's get started.

Background

Why Do I Pull Out my Eyelashes and Eyebrows?

Like me you might have never known before that when you pull your eyelashes and eyebrows out it's not just a quirky little habit you have, but a veritable medical condition. And you are not alone; thousands of people all over the world suffer from this very condition, known as 'hair pulling disorder, or 'Trichotillomania'.

What is Hair Pulling Disorder, or Trichotillomania?

Trichotillomania is classified as an impulse control disorder. People who suffer from this hair pulling disorder have the uncontrollable urge to pull out hair from their scalp, eyelashes, eyebrows or other parts of their body. Sufferers may have either general Trichtillomania where they pull out hair from all over the body, or a specific Trichotillomania where they pull out only certain types of hair, such as only eyelashes and eyebrows. Patients are unable to stop this behavior, even as their hair becomes thinner and results in noticeable bald patches. **It is more than just a nervous habit, which can be controlled through willpower or simply by deciding to stop.** This repetitive behavior is often self-destructive and distressing to the sufferer.

Most often patients pull hairs one-by-one, and often eat the hairs after plucking. Similar body focused-repetitive behaviors include skin picking, lip biting and nail biting. Despite the desire to stop harming their bodies in such a way, people who suffer from Trichotillomania have a hard time controlling these urges. This not only results in physical impairments but also significant emotional distress. **It is by no means a patient's fault for being unable to control such behavior.**

Trichotillomania is more than just a nervous habit, which can be controlled through willpower, or simply by deciding to stop

What Causes Eyelash Trichotillomania?

Research of causes and treatments of Trichotillomania are still in the early stages. Studies have shown evidence that indicates Trichotillomania to be a neurobiological disorder and may be linked to one's genetic makeup. Eyelash pulling is often triggered by stress, anxiety and depression. People with Eyelash Trichotillomania generally have a neurologically based, often genetic predisposition to pull their eyelashes as a self-soothing mechanism. 80% of eyelash pullers also report an itch-like urge to pull and there may well be a cause similar to folliculitis (inflammation of the hair root) or an irritation to the very natural and normal skin yeast, Malassezia.

However there is growing research that points to a multitude of causes, such as low Estrogen levels, a lack of certain minerals such as calcium and magnesium in the diet, serotonin deficiencies in the brain and traumatic childhood events. **Therefore it is very important for each individual to search for the treatment or combination of treatments that best suits his or her individual case.**

Eyelash pulling sessions are often carried out in a 'trance-like' state and the individual may 'wake up' to find themselves pulling their eyelashes or eyebrows without even realizing it. There are three main compulsions for eyelash pulling and it is important for the individual to work to recognize what 'motivation' causes them to pull in order for them to become completely self aware, a state that is essential for treatment (see section on self-awareness below):

- **Self-soothing**

  Many sufferers feel better when they pull because

pulling reduces other stimulation, allows the mind to focus on the act of pulling and thus the individual experiences a kind of soothing of the nervous system.

- ○ **<u>Stimulation</u>**

  Boredom can also be a culprit and pulling can provide the stimulation that the nervous system craves.

- ○ **<u>Perfectionism</u>**

  Sufferers of Trichotillomania may also be perturbed by the smallest imperfections and spend hours examining their eyelids and eyebrows trying to 'fix' them.

Eyelash pullers have a hard time controlling this obsessive-compulsive behavior due to the vicious cycle of complications that stems from Eyelash Trichotillomania. Eyelash pulling worsens the emotional instability that causes an individual to pull. Pulling momentarily satisfies a sufferer, but in the long run results in serious emotional consequences, such as severe self-consciousness, poor self-image, low self-esteem, fear of public places and other lifestyle setbacks. Individuals who pull tend to feel "freakish" or "crazy" because of the abnormal behavior and its effects.

We also recommend keeping a daily journal to pinpoint times when the urges seem more frequent or intense. You may find that these times are related to fluctuating hormone levels. If this is the case then you can prepare yourself for periods where you tend to be weaker. Forewarned is forearmed.

It is essential for each individual to find the cause and corresponding treatment or combination of treatments that best suits his or her personal needs.

Who Suffers from Eyelash Trichotillomania?

Trichotillomania is believed to affect 2-5% of the population and 80-90% of reported cases are women. The average age of onset is 11, however pulling can start at any age. Children under the age of 6 years old usually stop hair pulling after 12 months. **The condition affects all types of people from every different background. Eyelash pullers can range from very emotionally troubled, to otherwise quite healthy and successful people.** Sufferers are very often successful in other areas and have a difficult time understanding why they cannot control this aspect of their lives.

The diagnosis criteria for Eyelash Trichotillomania in the mental health field include a presence of multiple symptoms:

1. Eyelash pulling that results in noticeable hair loss

2. Relief and gratification during pulling

3. Increased tension when resisting pulling

4. Significant impairment in social functions due to pulling

Eyelash Trichotillomania affects many people from all different backgrounds. YOU ARE NOT ALONE.

The Phases of Eyelash Trichotillomania

There are three main phases to Eyelash Trichotillomania:

1. An initial experience of tension accompanied by a desire to pull out some eyelashes or eyebrows.

2. Eyelash pulling begins and feels good, with a sense of relief, as well as some excitement.

3. Once the eyelashes are pulled, the sufferer feels guilt, remorse, and shame. Attempts are made to cover the bald patches with makeup, eye pencils, eyeliner and sufferers begin hiding at this point, or to feel intensely humiliated.

Recognizing the phase you are in at any moment is an important first step to self awareness and eventually controlling your behavior.

Treatment

Unfortunately Eyelash Trichotillomania, along with many other obsessive-compulsive disorders such as skin picking is not very well understood. Because of the nature of the shame surrounding these conditions the true extent is misunderstood and thus the amount of research into these conditions is limited. Therefore, although there is growing research, there has not been conclusive evidence into which treatments work the best. In addition, because of the various causes for these behaviors, there are often many different types of therapy and treatment that will work. **This is why we recommend that sufferers try many different treatments in order to find those that work the best, and even better, that they often use many different methods simultaneously.**

There is no known 'cure' for Eyelash Trichotillomania but there are treatment options available. Discovering ways to control eyelash pulling impulses can help a patient become pull free. Cognitive behavior therapy, stress-control medications, and hair pulling support groups have all proven as an effective way to control symptoms. It is essential to understand that Eyelash Trichotillomania is a complex problem, and can have differing causes, so it may need to be approached from several different angles to find an effective treatment.

Therapy can help the sufferer become aware of the cycle of destructive thinking as well break this habitual thinking and responses.

Most importantly, belief is essential for those who suffer from Trichotillomania: to know that although it can be difficult to stop hair pulling, it IS POSSIBLE!

Cognitive Behavior Therapy

Cognitive Behavior Therapy is the primary treatment for eyelash pulling and trains patients in self-monitoring, identifying and responding to high-risk solutions, assessing the function of pulling, confronting realizations, and developing mindfulness. Basically it trains individuals to be aware of when and why they pull as a foundation to the treatment, and then helps sufferers find positive non-pull responses to these situations. It is founded on the theory that if you are fully aware of when and why you pull then you can find appropriate solutions.

There are various types of Cognitive Behavior Therapy, but perhaps the most popular of these is *Habit Reversal Training* (HRT). It's based on the thought that those that suffer from the condition pull their hair as a response to certain situations, contexts or occurrences. However these individuals are unaware of these triggers. So Habit Reversal

Training first teaches the individual how to understand the physical and emotional triggers that make them pull by being more aware of what is going on when they start to pull (the place, the events, the context, etc). Once these factors are understood, then the individual learns how to use other behaviors and coping strategies instead of eyelash pulling when these situations and events arise. These can include keeping the hands busy by squeezing a rubber ball or stroking on oil whenever the urge to pull arises.

Another very effective Cognitive Behavior Therapy method is known as *Mindfulness Based Cognitive Behavioral Therapy*. The objective with this therapy is to learn to accept certain experiences without judging them, no matter how uncomfortable they are. It is based on the theory that much of our suffering comes from trying to ignore, control or do away with unwanted feelings, emotions, thoughts and urges. What actually causes eyelash pulling is our efforts to ignore our problems rather than face them. Therefore the goal is to accept our difficult thoughts or experiences, without judging them and without pulling.

Other Cognitive Behavioral Therapy techniques that can be used alone or with other Cognitive Behavior Therapies methods are:

- o <u>Stimulus Control</u>

    Using actual items to block eyelash pullers from pulling by making it difficult for them to do so, as well as changing the environment to reduce the sensory input that causes pulling. For example, if a sufferer pulls whenever he looks in the mirror, then he should remove the mirror, or signal to himself not to go to the mirror with some sort of sign. Using glasses, gloves, fake fingernails or other items can prevent individuals from pulling. Or they can altogether avoid high-risk situations such as reading, working at the computer or watching television.

- ○ Cognitive Restructuring

  This method teaches sufferers to have different thought patterns when they feel an urge to pull. It is as if the individual were re-routing the neural pathways. An example would be to modify one's behaviors by stroking the area (with the use of an oil or cream for example) when an urge arises rather than pulling.

Cognitive Behavior Therapy is highly successful in many obsessive-compulsive cases and everyone should try this method.

Medication

Medications have proven less effective and more disappointing than behavioral therapy, and in general we discourage their use. There are several reasons for this:

o Most medications (Prozac, Clomipramine Anafranil, Fluoxetine, etc) affect the chemical Serotonin that is found in the brain. It is not known whether abnormal quantities or a shortage of serotonin is indeed a cause or an effect of eyelash pulling and other obsessive-compulsive disorders. Serotonin is said to have a role in regulating anxiety and its levels may be influenced by external factors, such as sunlight, diet and exercise. However findings have not been conclusive that this chemical is really responsible for eyelash pulling.

o   There are many side effects when taking these
    medications that can range in complexity and
    seriousness and may even exacerbate many
    obsessive-compulsive disorders.

o   Using medication that targets glutamate, a
    completely different chemical, has proven more
    beneficial (see following section on Amino Acids)
    than anti-depressants and other medications that
    affect Serotonin.

o   When researching various medical solutions it is
    important to consider the different interests
    involved. It is in the medical and pharmaceutical
    industries' best interest to encourage the use of
    costly medication. Natural and preventative remedies
    are rarely the first types of treatments that the
    established medical community will promote and

thus it is up to us, as individuals to find our own natural and holistic opportunities for healing.

o Because of the limited research or knowledge about these obsessive-compulsive disorders, many doctors are not educated enough in the possible treatments for these conditions. Therefore they may opt for what they see as the easiest solution. In my own and other's experiences, doctors often misdiagnose or are completely ignorant of these conditions.

o Individuals pull their eyelashes and eyebrows for many different reasons and may have different biological conditions to their pulling. Therefore a 'one size fits all' medication is most likely not to work.

We encourage individuals to look at what natural and 'alternative' treatments are available. **Due to our own and**

other's success, we strongly advocate a 'natural'
approach to healing, including modifications to diet,
exercise, awareness and mindfulness training,
homeopathy, using essential oils and behavior
modification therapy instead of pharmaceuticals and
medicating.

*Try a mixture of other therapies before embarking on a
purely medical solution.*

Amino Acids

Recently there has been much research into using the amino acid N-acetylcysteine (otherwise known as NAC) in the treatment of obsessive-compulsive conditions such as hair pulling, skin picking and nail biting. The results are heartening and NAC has been shown to greatly help in reducing urges, including those of hair pullers. According to the US National Library of Medicine and National Institute of Health, **"Fifty-six percent of patients were "much or very much improved" with N-acetylcysteine use compared with 16% taking placebo. Significant improvement was initially noted after 9 weeks of treatment."**

This is great news, not just because it is another tool in fighting Trichotillomania, but because positive results in studies like these encourage further research into the condition, which at the moment is rare. NAC affects the amount of glutamate in the brain, which causes excitement and can encourage pulling behavior.

N-acetylcysteine is an amino acid that can be bought online, in health food stores, or on our own site: http://trichotillomaniastop.com (see the end of this book for a special offer). For best results, any type of pharmaceutical therapy should be accompanied by some sort of Cognitive Behavior Therapy. If you do decide to use amino acids, make sure to talk to your doctor beforehand.

Amino Acids can be an effective part of an Eyelash Trichotillomania treatment program.

Consider Therapy

Consider starting therapy and getting professional help. While some individuals beat their obsessive-compulsive condition without it, there is no shame in getting professional help. Why reinvent the wheel after all? Get a therapist and take advantage of the wisdom and experience that has gone before you, as well as benefit from the contacts and resources that will become available to you. You would use an accountant, lawyer, doctor or other professional that is trained in their area for your other needs, so why not do the same for this very real condition that has such a big impact on your life?

Make sure that you research who you work with, however. Interview them to see what their approach is. Are they familiar with Trichotillomania? Do they overuse medical solutions? Do they use different methods or are they stuck in only one approach? Do they use 'alternative' treatments such as hypnosis and homeopathy, or are they only about prescribing 'meds'? Have a look on line and see if anyone is talking about the therapist in forums or have given reviews. **It is imperative to find the right fit for a therapist to be effective.**

Get professional help for this very real medical condition.

Living with Eyelash Pulling

Embracing Your Unique You

As difficult as it may seem, embracing your eyelash pulling as a part of your unique story is an important step forward. However you want to look at it, whether stemming from a lesson to be learned, something given to you to overcome, or just as genetic bad luck, it is important to see your condition as part of your life. **To accept your Eyelash Trichotillomania and to make peace with it.** Only then can you see it for what it is – a medical condition that you can treat- and then put together a system to beat, just as you would do with any other medical condition.

You may even want to see it as a challenge that you have been given to help you grow to be a stronger person. And perhaps one day, once you have conquered your eyelash pulling condition, you might turn around and help others with theirs.

Accept Eyelash Trichotillomania as a part of your own unique story.

Being an 'Ex' Eyelash Puller

It is essential to understand that someone who has quit pulling is an 'ex-puller' and will never be a 'non-puller'. I sometimes equate it to being an ex-smoker. That means eyelash pulling will always be a part of you and your history, and thus you will always have to remain self-aware and careful. Sometimes little urges will start to pop up and you will need to center yourself again. This situation will get easier to deal with over time, but it will never completely disappear. Therefore you must be conscious you have this weakness and be continuously mindful of it. While this might seem terribly heavy on your consciousness, it actually becomes easier and easier to cope with as you remain pull free. Soon it will merely be a fact that you are aware of, but that does not weigh too heavily.

Often admitting to others about your weakness and your status as an 'ex-puller' can help you remain strong by calling on them recognize your identity as well as to help you in certain moments of weakness.

It is vital to have a strategy prepared in case you do temporarily fall back into eyelash and eyebrow pulling patterns. **In these cases you must not get discouraged, but forgive yourself for your momentary weakness and deal constructively with the setback.**

Acknowledge and make peace with the fact that you are an 'ex-eyelash puller' and always will be.

Setbacks and How to Deal with Them

One word on setbacks: setbacks are a normal part of the process and you should be prepared for them. **Aim for gradual healing rather than a radical cold turkey approach, which will only cause frustration and loss of confidence.** Retraining the neural patterns as well as putting healing systems in place takes time, so allow yourself the time to heal. When you experience a setback, don't make a big deal out of it. Just pick yourself back up, dust yourself off, remember the gradual nature of recovery and start again. Understand that having been able to make any progress at all shows that it is possible. Now it just needs to become ingrained behavior, which it will, with enough time and practice.

Setbacks are normal and you should be prepared for them; most of all be kind to yourself.

Eyelash Pulling Tools

The Success Mindset: Using Visualization

The indispensible first step to getting the things that you want out of life is this: decide what you want. - Ben Stein

Visualization is a powerful tool that many successful athletes, businessmen and leaders use on a regular basis. It consists of picturing exactly what you want in order to help you get it. The practice has been the object of many studies and is based on the fact that your brain cannot recognize the difference between reality and imagination. So that if you imagine something often and clearly enough the brain will take it as truth and will do everything in its power to treat these visualizations as reality and help you achieve them.

Some guidelines for visualization:

- Be very clear with exactly what your vision is. See it in as much detail as possible. Include sounds, smells, and your emotions, with as much detail to make it real for your brain as possible. Imagine how you feel as you go out without any make up on, as someone compliments you on your beautiful eyes. Remember – you are programming your brain to achieve whatever you are picturing, so make it good.

- Visualize in an active, present tense. 'I am proud hearing a person compliment me on my beautiful eyelashes.' rather than 'I would be happy if..., or 'I am happy that I have beautiful thick lashes.', rather than 'When I don't have any more bald patches I will be happy...'.

- When a negative thought comes in to quash your vision isolate the thought, turn it into black and white, cut the sound off, reduce it to a speck and then imagine blowing the negative thought away.

- Visualize on a daily basis. When you get up in the morning and before you go to sleep. Consider putting together a vision board, full of images and quotes that will inspire you when you contemplate it.

- Include every detail in your life, not just your hair pulling goals. Imagine the house you live in, the holidays you take, the time you spend with your kids, a full life like you want to live it.

- Remember - the sky is the limit. The more you wish for, the more you will get. If you can't even imagine success, then it is sure that it will elude you.

- Fill out a chart like this to get started. Be sure each goal is measurable, detailed and has a time limit.

Relations	Financial	Professional	Eyelash Pulling	Personal

Time and again visualization has been proven a valuable free resource, so tap into it.

Auto-hypnosis

Using auto-hypnosis can help you conquer that part of you that is working against your own best interest and harness the power of your own mind to beat Eyelash Trichotillomania. **Consciously, you may know all the good reasons not to pull, but you need to feel, not just think, differently about pulling your eyelashes and eyebrows out.** The basic thing to know about auto-hypnosis is that the mind is most receptive when it is calm and the body is relaxed. So the key to success in autohypnosis is simply relaxing the body and quieting the mind.

Follow this 10-step process to use autohypnosis as a part of your Trich cure:

1. Develop the suggestion that you will use during your auto-hypnosos. It must be

   o positive, with no negative words.

- o short, between 6 and 15 words.

- o meaningful, this is what you really want to happen.

- o possible, something you can achieve. Avoid absolutes and time limits.

- o focused, tackle one suggestion at a time, not many different wishes.

- o For example "Every day I do not pull out any eyelashes."

2. Write your suggestion on a piece of paper

- o in clear, neat handwriting.

- o write as if you were writing to your best friend or lover.

- o concentrate and write slowly thinking about the meaning of the words as you write each of them.

- o Repeat the message to yourself, preferably out loud, listening carefully to yourself, and to your words. Think clearly about their meaning.

3. Find a place where you can relax and be by yourself. You might put on some of your favorite music in the background (no singing).

4. You should carry out the auto-hypnosis programming three times a day:

   o When you wake up in the morning - as soon as possible after awakening.

   o In the middle of the day, best just after lunch.

   o Just before going to sleep at night

5. Sit or lie comfortably and find something to look at and focus on. Take three deep breaths, letting yourself relax all over and feeling the stress and tension leaving your body with each exhalation. Breathe in serenity, breathe out tension.

6. Close your eyes and hold the last breath for at least 10

seconds then slowly let it all out, letting all the tension in all of your muscles flow outward with that last exhalation.

7. Now that you are relaxed, and breathing evenly and smoothly, begin to count backwards from 5 to 1. As you count you feel yourself relaxing deeper and deeper with each and every breath you take, with every number you count.

8. When you reach the count of 1, feel yourself drop quickly and deeply into a very comfortable and relaxed state of mind.

9. Now begin to say, in your mind, not out loud, the words you wish to program into your subconscious, repeating the phrase 20 times. To help you keep count, each time you say the phrase, move the tip of a finger to the tip of your thumb. Do not hurry. Go slow and deep. After you

have mastered the process, it becomes automatic and you don't have to pay too much attention to either the hand movements or the words themselves. This might take a few days.

10. As you improve, begin to focus on relaxing deeper and deeper, drifting away, just letting yourself completely relax. Don't rush the process. When you find yourself able to think of other things, begin to parallel the suggestion with the following thoughts:

   o "Each and every word you hear me say takes you deeper and deeper into a very beneficial state of relaxation."

   o "You can hear my words giving you suggestions, these suggestions will make your life better and happier."

   o "Each and every time I do this exercise the effect is

stronger and more beneficial. The suggestion is helping improve my life more and more as I move deeper and deeper during the exercises."

Hypnosis can help you prepare your mind and affect changes in your behavior.

Coming Around the Problem

This method is what I call 'Coming around the problem'. What I mean by this is when you step back and look at the context of your eyelash pulling, when you look at the rest of your life and analyze where you can make other changes, it will not only put your eyelash and eyebrow pulling into perspective, but it will give you other areas to focus on. **Setting goals in other areas of your life and making improvements in completely unrelated parts of your life will give you a sense of accomplishment which will boost confidence and will lay the foundations for success in the more complex areas such as eyelash pulling.** By starting on small changes to improve your life you will put the basics in place to start feeling more confident and happy. And success breeds success. Take, for example, the case outlined in Charles Duhigg's best selling book 'The Power of Habit' (a recommended read – see our

'Recommended Resources' section). By changing her exercise habits and daily living patterns the individual at the beginning of the book managed to stop smoking. Work on building a better life one brick at a time and starting with small, easy to succeed tasks and the next thing you know you're whole life will transform. Not only do you treat your eyelash pulling, but you also transform your life. What a very heartening and exciting proposition!

Work on living a happy, fulfilling life rather than narrowly obsessing with your eyelash and eyebrow pulling.

8 Step Trich Stop System

This 8 step system is a proven system for helping you to stop eyelash pulling, no matter how long you have been pulling. These 7 steps, along with the tools above will help you put in place an effective plan for your successful Trich cure.

1. Before you begin

Be kind to yourself. You are not alone and you are not a freak. Eyelash Trichotillomania is a legitimate condition that you suffer from. You can beat it, but it is hard, so be kind with yourself as you move through the system. If you slip and do pull don't berate yourself, just accept that it is a part of the cure and get back on the plan. I often compared myself to my husband who was quitting smoking, and tried to be as kind and understanding to myself as I was with him. It's TOUGH, but YOU CAN DO IT.

2. Recognize The Condition

Acknowledge that you have a problem. The first thing to realize is that you suffer from treatable disorder, not something due to willpower or lack thereof. The disorder arises as a result of genetic makeup, moods, and your background and is a condition in need of treating, not something to beat yourself up over. On the other hand, don't convince yourself that nothing is wrong. Eyelash Trichotillomania can be considered a form of self-harm, and like all forms of self-harm, eyelash pulling can become an addictive behavior, so you need to recognize and treat it as such. My big breakthrough was when I finally realized that my pulling was a legitimate condition. This freed me of guilt and shame and allowed me to move forward to looking for the treatment that best suited me and my own personal version of the condition.

3. Identify When You Pull

Know your triggers. Eyelash pulling becomes addictive because of the natural pain-killing 'buzz' that self-harm gives us; the body's natural morphine kicks in. When do you pull your eyelashes and eyebrows out? In the evening when watching television? When speaking to your annoying mother in law on the phone? When reading or working on the computer? Make a list of your triggers and next to each write down an alternative activity that would make you feel better in these contexts.

The initial cause of Eyelash Trichotillomania could be genetic and/or environmental, and researchers see similarities with the triggers for obsessive-compulsive disorder. Distressing childhood experiences or disturbed early relationships with parents might be behind the development of this disorder, and one study has shown that over two-thirds of sufferers have experienced at least one traumatic event in their lives, with a fifth of them diagnosed with post-traumatic stress disorder. This has led researchers to believe that it may be a way to cope for some sufferers. Therefore in your own case, regardless of what may or may not have brought on the condition, consider what kinds of situations cause you to resort to eyelash pulling. Do you only do it when you're depressed? Angry? Confused? Frustrated? Bored? Once you identify and understand what triggers your eyelash pulling, you can find other, more positive ways of coping.

4. Write Down When You Pull and Keep a Journal

Keep a journal or a chart of your pulling episodes. Through writing you can get a good idea of the times, the triggers, and the impact of your eyelash pulling. Record the date, time, location, and number of eyelashes or eyebrows you pull and what you used to pull them. Write down your thoughts or feelings when you pull as well. This is a good way of relieving yourself of the guilt and shame, and of expressing how the eyelash pulling is impacting your life in general. You will begin to identify your weak moments and mental states. By being more aware of these moments and feelings you will begin to master them. You may be surprised to see how many eyelashes you have pulled or how much time you have spent doing so. You may also be surprised to find times that you pull that you were not aware of, or feelings that reoccur. You will also want to use a journal to express your emotions. Write out a list of the consequences you've experienced as a result of your eyelash pulling. It might include comments from people you have endured, or having to go to great lengths with eyeliner. It should also include the relationship consequences, such as not going on a date or to spending time with people because you're afraid they will find out about your eyelash pulling.

5. Make a Plan

Develop a 'Recognize, Interrupt, and Alternatives Plan' to help you stop pulling your eyelashes and eyebrows out. This consists of noticing when you feel like pulling and then interrupting the feelings and urges by listening to visualization and positive reminders in your head. Then, choose an alternative action, something that will relax you or deal with the feelings that bring on the compulsion to pull. Alternative ways of expressing your emotions and might be deep breathing and clearing your mind, rehearsing your visualization, drawing or writing, calling a friend that knows about your condition or not, beginning a manual activity such as beading, needlepoint or video games. Many people have found using physical reminders effective, such as wearing weights that pull on the arms, gloves or fake fingernails as a reminder and a hindrance to pulling.

6. Keep An All Natural Oil Close at Hand

Using an all natural oil, such The Trich Stop Hairgrowth Oil (

for more information:

http://trichotillomaniastop.com/hair-growth-oil/) was the

absolute key to my success to stop pulling my eyelashes and

eyebrows out. It has been specially developed to calm and

sooth your follicles as well as stimulate re-growth. I

developed it as an aid to help me with my own condition and

would use it whenever I had an urge to pull as an alternative

action. I suffered from itchy, irritated follicles and the serum

was a relief for the 'physical' and uncomfortable sensation

pushing me to pull. In addition the oiliness made it difficult

to pull and it was a comfort that I was nourishing the hair

follicles and encouraging re-growth. Keep your oil with you

at times that you are susceptible to pull and choose it as an

alternative action as well as a soother and a reminder that

you are experiencing your triggers and that you can overcome them. (see the end of this book for a special reader offer).

7. Find What Works For You

Every Eyelash Trichotillomania suffer is different. Use the Trich Stop System to put a personalized plan in place for your own eyelash pulling condition. You will want to experiment with different steps of the process to identify what is the most effective for you.

8. Use Auxiliary Activities

Do not skip using the auxiliary activities such as visualization and auto-hypnosis. They are powerful tools and in conjunction with the Trich Stop System will be sure to lead you to beating eyelash pulling successfully!

Trich Stop Top Tips

These tips in conjunction with the Trich Stop Steps will help you beat eyelash pulling!

Systems and Structures Are The Key

Do not leave your treatment to chance. Put in place concrete structures and a plan to eliminate the chaos in your life and give you guidelines and a context as support. This is key to success. As we have mentioned before, by making even the slightest changes in other areas of your life you can have an effect on your eyelash pulling actions. You don't have to be extremely rigid. If you have a party to attend, and can't follow your routine, that's ok. You can be flexible, but just give yourself a framework to work within.

In addition, change your lifestyle habits and you will interrupt the underlying patterns of your eyelash pulling action. For example, if you know that you have weak moments in the evening as you sit in front of the television, then choose another activity at that time – take a walk, exercise, practice a musical instrument. If you find yourself spending hours in front of the mirror after your evening shower then start taking it in the morning when you don't have time and have to get out the door to work.

By both putting some skeletal structures in place, and shaking up your daily routine you will create a winning atmosphere for your treatment.

If You Slip Up

Do not beat yourself up over any slip-ups. This will happen and is a natural part of the process. Just use the mistake as a learning experience to better understand your eyelash pulling and continue to develop the best solution for your personal version of the condition.

Write down your mistakes in your journal, try to understand why they occurred and suggest to yourself possible solutions. Use these slips as a chance to learn more about your own personal condition. **Remember, true success is having control over your behaviors that will lead to less and less eyelash pulling episodes**. Your goal should not be to go cold turkey, which could cause unbearable frustration that will lead to certain relapse, but to gradually pull less and less in a structured way, with pulling episodes becoming less frequent so that one day you wake up and you haven't pulled for a very long time!

See slip-ups as a learning experience and keep at it; healing is a gradual process.

Successfully Identify Trigger Times

Of course, sometimes you will find yourself pulling out your eyelashes without even having been aware of any triggers (although there is always one). So you might want to use something to physically help identify your trigger times, such as weights on your arms during danger times when you might become in a trancelike state and not realize your pulling activity (such as speaking on the phone, watching television, reading or working on your computer).

You might also realize that certain situations, or the lead up to these moments, are a trigger for you. Perhaps confronting an estranged relative, speaking to your boss or attending a social event alone causes stress that then manifests itself in eyelash pulling. **By understanding these causes better you can put steps in place that will allow you to recognize the danger, become more self-aware and** allow you to create a different mental picture of how these moments can play out.

By understanding your personal triggers (not every hair pullers are the same) you will become self-aware and can put in place alternative actions and responses to the situations and the lead up to eyelash pulling.

Use Distraction

Get into the habit of doing something else when you get the urge to pull, such as going for a walk, doing needlepoint, writing in your journal, etc. **Distraction isn't just about doing something else, it's about retraining the brain to the point where it starts to feel more natural not to pull in response to your trigger times.**

In addition by using distracting activities you will begin to reorganize your life, bringing positive influences to play. Analyze the way you spend your time. Are you watching too much TV or leading a solitary life? Are you spending enough time exercising or with friends? Do you spend too much time on Facebook, comparing yourself to others, sure that they have a better life than you (research has indicated that people who spend a lot of time on Facebook are less happy than those that don't)?

In order to use distraction for the most benefit, try different hobbies and find an activity that makes your heart sing. One that you can spend your time doing, which will bring you happiness and confidence, while allowing your hands to lose themselves by doing something else rather than pulling. It doesn't really matter what the activity is, or how well you do it, as long as you enjoy it. Hobbies such as jewelry making, collecting stamps, or learning car mechanics are a constructive way to use your time. Or exercise activities like dance, Tai Chi, or other sports will give you the perfect distraction. Take a class to learn a new language or more about Art History. There are a multitude of activities and hobbies to try, and one is sure to take your fancy.

Think about something you have always wanted to do and order a book about it on Amazon. Or even better, sign up for a class at a local cultural center or community college. Not only will this give you a source of distraction, it can help you begin to make small changes in your daily life that will lead to big changes in your eyelash pulling condition.

Besides distraction, an activity or hobby will give you confidence, a fresh outlook and the possibility to meet new people.

Use Natural Oils and Aromatherapy

Organic oils (such as castor, olive and jojoba) and herbs (such as rosemary, thyme, lavender) can be used daily to help reduce the urge to pull, and also help your follicles heal and eyelashes grow. They will also make the eyelashes oily and difficult to pull.

In addition these essences have a calming influence on the psyche and can relieve tension and stress.

Using nature's own medicine is used for many different conditions in many countries that have leading healthcare. In Europe olive oil is even used to treat diaper rash!

Use all natural products to soothe your follicles, treat your Trichotillomania and encourage eyelash and eyebrow growth.

Consider Getting a Pet

If you like animals then consider getting a pet. Much research has shown that animals can be a positive part of many types of therapy. **Pets have been shown to reduce stress and make people happier in general.**

Having a pet is has many upsides. Firstly, it gives you an activity that will both serve as distraction and allow you to meet new people. Taking your dog for a walk or to a dog park will not only make exercising fun and easy, but it will give you the chance to meet other dog owners. When you feel an urge coming on you can grab the brush and give your cat a good combing. Not only will this serve as distraction and keep your hands busy, but grooming animals is a proven stress reliever.

Taking care of your pet also gives you a sense of kindness and responsibility as well as achievement.

Lastly, and certainly most importantly, animals are a source of unconditional love like no other.

An animal will give you love, comfort and an activity to keep you busy.

Mirror, Mirror, on the Wall...

Stop looking in the mirror! Examining the area will only focus your attention on it and your failure to control yourself. This includes even after you have pulled to see the damage. Eyelash pullers often report suddenly finding themselves in a trancelike state in front of the mirror, sometimes not even remembering how they got there. In order to avoid this, remove any bedside mirrors and put a sign on any other mirrors in the house reminding yourself to stop. Or place notes on the way (the bathroom door for example) instructing yourself to not continue any further. Turn down the lights when you are in the bathroom so that you cannot get a good look in the mirror when you are there.

If you have confided in a family member have them help you with gentle reminders or distraction if they see you heading towards a mirror.

This is also a perfect time to just apply an all natural oil in order to retrain your neural pathways, ignore the area and the next thing you know, when you do catch a glimpse of yourself, SURPRISE, you'll have hair growth instead of bald patches!

It seems like such a simple thing to do, but stopping oneself from looking in the mirror constantly can be one of the major keys to peace of mind and success.

Watch your diet

Having a healthy body is key to laying the foundations to successfully beat Trich and grow your eyelashes back. There are many studies that show that nutrition can contribute to exacerbating urges to pull. **In addition, having a healthy body and feeling good about yourself will create the positive, confident feeing that you need to underscore a successful treatment.**

Cut out processed foods, eat a balanced healthy diet and exercise when you can. Exercise improves circulation throughout your body, including your scalp, which can result in faster eyelash growth and soothed follicles. **Eat the foods that your body needs to beat Trich, keep hair follicles healthy and grow thick, strong eyelashes back quickly:**

· Vitamin A is essential for hair growth. Natural food sources include mango, orange, carrot, sweet potato, and squash. But don't take supplements as too much can actually cause hair loss.

· Vitamin B boosts the production of hemoglobin, which helps follicles receive enough oxygen to stay healthy and promote hair growth. Eat potatoes, garbanzo beans/chickpeas, chicken breast, oatmeal, pork loin, and roast beef.

· Potassium. The highest concentrations are found in bananas and the added potassium helps to balance out deficiencies that can contribute to eyelash pulling urges.

· Folic acid is found in collard greens, lentils, garbanzo beans/chickpeas, papaya, peas, and asparagus, folic acid contributes to natural hair regrowth.

· Vitamin E also helps blood circulate and improve eyelash growth and can be found in most cereals, almonds, safflower oil, corn oil, and soybean oil.

· Vitamin C is required for the development of collagen, which is necessary for growing strong hair. Eat kiwi fruit, guava, red peppers, and oranges.

· Try using herbal supplements such as Valerian root, Passionflower or St John's Wort. These are often used as natural tranquilizers and can be used as a calming medication.

· Green tea contains theanine, an amino-acid which is a mood enhancer and reduces stress. It also lowers blood pressure, helps brain functions and has many other positive effects on health. To get the most benefit, make sure to use whole leaves and follow the instructions for making the tea carefully (teabags and over boiled tea lose their healthy properties.

· Make sure to get enough potassium, calcium, zinc and magnesium. Deficiencies of these minerals have been linked to obsessive-compulsive disorders, including studies where cows that have abnormally low levels of these minerals

chew on their skin and pull out their hair.

A balanced and healthy diet will give you confidence and

help you heal from the inside out.

Avoid Chemicals

Whether in your diet, in your household cleaning supplies, as a part of medication or in your cosmetics, reduce the chemicals that are present in your daily life. Life today is replete with chemicals that are brandished as the cure for everything from runny noses to dog smells in the carpet. However the presence of these chemicals can be harmful in discreet ways. Current research is beginning to show that over exposure to common chemicals can be more harmful than previously thought. Some everyday products are now suspected to have a role in increasing rates of diseases like cancer as well a behavioral conditions such as autism.

This includes cosmetics. Do not use heavily chemical creams, makeup, or eyeliners as this can be irritating, preventing healing and actually causing you to have more urges.

Only use all natural products such as essential oils and herbal essences, and reduce the presence of chemicals in your daily routine.

Using Makeup

For eyelash and eyebrow pulling, while it's incredibly tempting to hide behind makeup, ideally you should use as little as possible. Makeup exacerbates the problem, doesn't encourage healing and causes you to spend your energy on analyzing the results of your eyelash pulling as you put it on.

This is especially the case for false eyelashes. The adhesive irritates the follicles causing more urges and can even damage the follicles causing permanent hair loss. **When you are at home or with your family and friends try forgoing makeup.**

Of course there are times when you will want to wear makeup. In this case use a light, organic eyeliner or eyebrow pencils. If you must use makeup, then make sure it is composed of natural ingredients and use as little as possible.

This includes once you have control over your condition. I often long to wear mascara in order to show off the lashes that I have worked so hard to regrow. However I know that the chemicals will aggravate the follicles, and the added attention and irritation to the area will tempt my condition to return. Therefore, as frustrating as it is, I completely avoid using any makeup on my eyes.

Avoid false eyelashes, only use all natural make up, or even better, try going without.

Give Homeopathy a Try

Homeopathy can be an effective aid in helping control eyelash and eyebrow pulling. While little known in the US, many countries promote homeopathy both as a preventative medicine and an active cure. In fact, in countries where medical treatment is paid for by the government, homeopathy is actively promoted and paid for in order to keep medical costs down. France, for example, reimburses preventative and curative homeopathic treatments.

Homeopathic therapy is surprisingly effective in rebalancing a sufferer's mental, emotional, and physical well being, which will help in long term treatment of eyelash pulling. Homeopathic cures are successfully used to treat anxiety, phobias and panic attacks, influencing the patient's moods and assisting in stopping compulsive eyelash pulling behavior. It works as a stimulus, breaking the trance and helping the puller to shift his or her attention. Homeopathic remedies have also shown impressive results in helping patients see themselves as confident individuals. **Homeopathic treatment is a curative, non-toxic, gentle and modern treatment.** As it works in conjunction with the person's own internal drive towards equilibrium and healing, it influences brain chemistry and helps the patient gain in psychological strength. Homeopathic treatment is based on the idea that body and mind are dynamically interconnected and that both directly influence each other, and thus both must be treated for effective results.

To put in place your own homeopathic therapy, either seek out a homeopathic counselor to put together a personalized treatment, or put together your own by researching the various options. Many natural treatments are available as an aid to support other methods in the fight against the urges that cause hair pulling. Bach Flower remedies, for example can aid in calming the emotions while dealing with any underlying issues. This preparation includes agrimony, beech, cherry plum, white chestnut, chestnut bud, and others calming plants. Additional treatment options include St John's Wort, Valerian root, and Passion flower.

Create your own a homeopathic treatment to influence your brain and lay down a positive foundation for healing.

Exercise

Exercise has many different positive effects on those suffering from obsessive-compulsive disorders such as Eyelash Trichotillomania. Exercise boosts levels of serotonin, a chemical in the brain that is often a culprit in obsessive-compulsive disorders. While not completely understood, working to rebalance the brain has been known to reduce impulsive actions such as eyelash pulling. **The age-old philosophy teaches us that the way to a fulfilling and happy life is having a healthy brain in a healthy body.** Much like a 'runner's high', exercise routines are known to stimulate the brain, produce endorphins and make the individual 'feel good'. Often this stimulus can replace the stimulus that pulling gives, as well as relieving the tension that often comes before a pulling session. As you continue to exercise both the results you see, and the positive feelings produced when exercising, will increase your self confidence and self discipline. This will start you on an upward spiral of positive reinforcement.

As an added bonus, exercise improves circulation throughout your body, which can result in faster healing and eyelash and eyebrow growth.

You can also use it as a distraction when you are feeling an urge coming on or when you need to find a replacement activity for trigger times. While it may be difficult to get motivated, don't stress by thinking that you have to join a gym, be a member of a team or practice in public. Start with small steps such as taking a walk when you are susceptible to pull, and use it as an important part of your habit reversal training. Once you start feeling more confident you can choose any number of other sports that can be carried out either in a team or as an individual, such as swimming, BMX, skiing, horseback riding, or skating. Who knows, once you start seeing some progress you can even join a local league

to help you feel less isolated.

A healthy mind in a healthy body is one of the foundations

for a balanced and happy life.

The Benefits of Yoga, Meditation and Breathing Exercises

Yoga and meditation are not only natural ways to deal with stress, but they are the perfect mix of spiritual and bodily health.

Meditate regularly, once a day. The calming benefits of mediation spill over into the rest of your day. Aim to meditate at the same time everyday, whether in the morning, afternoon or evening. You can also use meditation in your habit reversal training, meditating to clear your mind whenever you get an urge, or find yourself in the process of pulling.

Choose a spot that is calm and comfortable, starting with just a few minutes with the long term goal to getting to 30 minutes. The objective of your meditation should be to clear your mind. You can use breathing techniques, such as concentrating on feeling your breathing going in and out, or you can try a tape or guided meditation. Simply concentrating on each breath as it goes in and out is a powerful way to promote inner peace. Use your diaphragm when you breathe and paradoxically, push your stomach out when you breathe in and vice versa when breathing out. Simply focus on your breathing and how it feels, eliminating any worries or thoughts, allowing your mind to quiet and be perfectly in the present. In the beginning your mind will continually try and break into your thoughts, but just keep bringing it back to your breathing and the here and now.

Patience and daily practice will help you get more comfortable with an 'empty' mind that will bring you peace. This is what is known as controlling 'the monkey mind', or the inner you that repeats limiting and negative thoughts. The monkey mind might continually tell you how ugly your hair is, or focus on bald spots. Using meditation will also help you clear out any bottled up emotions, freeing you from that stress. Using this method will teach you self-discipline and how to block your thoughts from a frantic mind.

You may also find yoga helpful as a sort of active meditation. Yoga is an age-old practice that signifies linking the body and mind. It is a great tool for helping you with mindfulness and breathing techniques can help you stop and focus on what is going on in your head. It will allow you to stretch your body, opening up your psyche and making you feel refreshed and less stressed. This will limit the anxiety that can often lead to urges to pull. To begin practicing yoga, while being taught the basics by a competent teacher is important, don't let this create a barrier for you. Other than finding a class in your area, you can begin by using a DVD, consult a book or even watch online videos.

In this same vein you can try alternatives such as Tai Chi or Qi Gong. These practices allow you to slow your movements down and allow you to become 100% conscious of your actions. Learning how to be conscious of your actions can help you with consciousness when pulling. Slowing down your actions, your thoughts and speech can give you a chance to focus on what is really going on and becoming mindful.

For any of these activities you must practice them regularly and for a period of time before seeing the results, so stick with it and don't just give up within a few days of beginning.

The link between body and mind fostered in yoga and mediation can lay solid foundations for a successful Eyelash Trichotillomania treatment.

Accept, Forgive and Let Go

Accept the past and any experiences that could lead to your anxiety and then, instead of dwelling on them, let go of the past. **Let go of the regrets, the fear, the anxiety and live in the now.** While easier said than done, this is an important step towards long term healing. There are no many studies that say that over analysis in therapy can actually cause more harm than good by reinforcing the negative messaging that is imprinted in your brain. Recent research is showing that finding the source of emotional instability is important, but then instead of picking at it and analyzing it over and over again it is best to acknowledge it and then let it go. To recognize that that was then and this is now and each individual controls his own destiny.

If there are individuals in your past that have done you harm, either knowingly or not, recognize the harm, forgive and then let go. As hard as it may be, do not harbor grudges, point fingers, or blame others for your current situation. **Know that you are powerful and can change your life and your now.** Actually, no one can change it but you, so accept this responsibility and challenge with open arms.

Allow your mind to focus on the good and positive. When it wanders into the negative bring it back and focus on the good solutions that your mind produces for any problems. Listen to your intuition and be kind to yourself. Let go of things that might have happened to you that you cannot control. **Train yourself to focus only on the things that you can control and that will make a difference in your life today.**

Today is the first day of the rest of your life.

Choose Happiness

This may seem very simplistic, but your state of mind is very often a choice. **Happiness is not just a state, but an actual DECISION.** It is surprising the difference that just a simple active decision to choose happiness will make.

Deciding to be happy starts with understanding that it is the smallest things in life that make us truly happy. It may be trite and it may be old fashioned, but it's true. Stopping to savor a beautiful sunset, a good laugh with an old friend over coffee, a moment of quiet to read your book are truly the secret to a happy life.

Stop comparing yourself to others, or looking for great events to happen to bring you 'happiness', but be grateful everyday for the small moments of contentment. When you add these up you will realize that happiness, no matter what your condition, is indeed within your grasp.

Happiness is a decision.

Try a Hypnotist

While hypnotism has a reputation for gold chains and clucking like a chicken, medical hypnosis is regaining credibility in the medical field as an important part of treatment for certain conditions including addictions and obsessive-compulsive disorders. **Hypnosis actually creates a hyper alert state, allowing the subconscious to be highly open to suggestion.** In fact, David Speigel from Stanford University has been able to show the impact of hypnosis on the brain, allowing for the effects to be measured scientifically.

This book gives you the tools for auto-hypnosis (see section on auto-hypnosis), which is an effective tool for you to use on your own. However it is worth looking into having hypnosis carried out by a professional as part of your continued treatment.

Using the powerful suggestive affects of hypnosis has been proven to help in obsessive-compulsive disorders.

A Mental Shift

Belief in the ability to change your habits and your life is more important than you know. **The mind can determine how the body functions and ultimately your future.** Take for example Dr Roger Bannister, the man who ran the first four-minute mile in the 1950's. People had said that it was an unbreakable barrier, but within a year or so of Dr. Bannister's feat, some 30 other runners had done the same. The world hadn't suddenly produced a new breed of super athletes, but Dr. Bannister's astonishing feat had changed the mindset of many runners. Instead of saying 'That's impossible' they were now saying 'I could do that'. And this mental shift impacted how their body performed.

Much as is used in the Alcoholics Anonymous program, this same 'power of the mind' can be used in a treatment program for Eyelash Trichotillomania.

Use Natural Stress Reducers

Incorporate more stress reducers in your life such as getting regular massages, having a pet or spending more time with the one that you have, listening to soothing music, or doing simple pleasant chores such as gardening.

Make a list of the things that bring you joy (use the 'Personal Stress Reducers' page in the Workbook) and refer to it when you begin to feel stress or anxiety coming on. Choose an activity and throw yourself into it to avoid falling into a negative mindset or increasing the tension in your life.

Activities can be either active (playing a sport or instrument, taking a walk, needlepoint, painting, dancing) or passive (listening to music, having a massage, etc), but should bring you no strings attached enjoyment. If playing a sport will give you stress because you need to be with people or practicing your guitar will put the pressure on because you really should practice more, then try another activity. This should be a moment of pure pleasure.

Enjoy your life!

Act NOW

Picasso was right, action IS the key to success. Take action now, even if it is a small step forward. A little bit everyday will set you on the path and make it easy to make progress every day. Don't just do this for your eyelash pulling condition. Do this for every part of your life. As you move forward, the better you will feel about your accomplishments, and the more self confidence you will obtain.

"Action is the key to success." – Pablo Picasso

About Spirituality

Everyone has a different version of spirituality, and whether you believe in putting yourself in God's hands or prefer to look within, having some kind of contact with your own spirituality is an important step for embracing who you are. **You need to find an inner peace, and whatever works for you, whether it's organized religion or individual spirituality, just make sure that it is based on loving yourself.** Whether it's a program similar to the spiritual based 12 step Alcoholic Anonymous program, or just open discussion between individuals with similar outlooks, there are many people who rely on prayer, meditation and getting in touch with their spiritual side to help them through certain obsessive compulsive behaviors. Carry out these activities on your own, or find individuals with a similar outlook either in your community or on the Internet.

Exploring your own personal spirituality can strengthen the foundations of your Eyelash Trichotillomania treatment.

Tricks

While an underlying system change is required and the traditional 'tricks' such as keeping your hands busy, etc aren't a long lasting cure, they can help you to slow down enough to think about what you are doing and give you an alternative action. These tricks can also be used as part of your Cognitive Behavior Treatment as Stimulus Control.

The following are some that other readers and followers of the Trich Stop System have sent in:

o Wear interesting earrings that you can play with. One parent we know even allowed their son to pierce his ears in order to get give him something other than hair to play with. The mother told me that this was 'thinking outside the box.'

o Program yourself to press your fingers together (or 'push the button') instead of pulling whenever you feel a trigger. This will gradually retrain your brain's reaction to triggers.

o Keep fingernails trimmed at all times to make it difficult to grab hold of the eyelash

o Try acrylic false nails which make it difficult to pull

o Wear glasses (even if they are fake!) which will create a barrier to your eyelashes and eyebrows and will give you more confidence in public

o Set up alarm reminders on your telephone or computer for the times when you most often pull. Make the title of the reminder something encouraging, a positive message to yourself such as 'YOU are in control', 'Don't Pull' or 'Go pet the cat'

o Use an all natural oil to reprogram your brain to stroke your follicles rather than pull

- Put up inspirational and kind notes to yourself around the house. Don't just give yourself commands, but send yourself positive affirmations such as 'I am worthy of love.' Or 'I deserve to have nice eyelashes.'

- Go to sleep early and get up early. Besides making you 'healthy, wealthy and wise' you will have less time to ponder, fret, and pull.

If you have any ideas you'd like to share with others then why not send us your ideas for our next edition of 'Eyelash Pulling' or our website?

Dealing with Others

One of the hardest parts of being a eyelash puller is dealing with the social implications, whether it is social situations, meeting new people or explaining the conditions to friends and family.

Don't Isolate Yourself

As much as you may want to hide away, isolation will only cause you more pain, stress and set the stage for eyelash pulling. This does not mean that you have to go to parties or speak in public. However do not refuse all social interaction. Start slowly. Choose a few friends or family members and confide in them. Tell them that you need their help. Go out with one or two people for short periods.

Church or religious groups can also be a supportive and understanding atmosphere to cultivate friendships. Join a group specific for hair pulling, or more general obsessive-compulsive disorders, or if you cannot find any in your area, join an online group.

Consider going to conferences such as those held by the Trichotillomania Learning Center where you can meet those suffering from similar issues.

No man is an island.

Go Online, Use Forums and Don't Be Afraid to Reach Out for Help!

Use the online (and offline) support groups that are available. However, be judicious when choosing the one you will participate in. Try out several and give them a chance until you find the one that matches your personal style. **Be careful to choose a support group that is positive, believes in a cure and is looking to help you in your success, not one that is full of complainers and moaners and people that just want to commiserate together.** Those kinds of groups will surely fail as they have already decided to fail in their minds. Remember eyelash pulling is a condition and so you need the right mental state to beat it. A positive outlook is key, so surround yourself with positive people. Having a group of successful people helping others overcome their condition is one of the keys strengths of organizations such as Alcoholics Anonymous. Recreate this same type of situation for yourself by choosing a positive support group that has people that have successfully beat Eyelash Trichotillomania.

By surrounding yourself with winners you too will become a winner.

Avoid Negative People and Cut Dead Wood

Avoid people that make you feel envious, silly or bad about yourself. Even family members or old friends. If they bring you down, then cut them out of your life. Surround yourself with people that bring you up. Also cut out worriers or doom and gloom people. Those that feel sorry for themselves, or for you.

Consider the effect that social media has on your life. Does Facebook make you feel bad about yourself? Do you spend your time comparing yourself to others? Does your online Trichotillomania group complain and moan? Do the books that you read about your condition belabor the negative emotions and put no constructive message out there?

It is a known fact that you are like the people that you surround yourself with. Your parents were right when they told you to pick the right type of friends. So begin today by making sure that everyone you have contact with loves you, supports you unconditionally, believes in you and has a bright, positive outlook. After all, you deserve only the best people in your life!

Cutting out any negative influence and surrounding yourself with a positive vibe will have a lasting impact on your success.

Family and Friends: Talk About Your Condition and Ask for Help

While you may be tempted to keep your condition in the dark, choose a few people to confide in. This may seem like a daunting prospect, but it is essential to put aside the shame. By opening up to a friend or loved one, not only will you feel less isolated, but you can call on the person to help you in various ways, whether it be reminding you not to look in the mirror, being 'on call' so that you can contact them when you need distraction or are feeling a need to pull, helping you stay on track with your treatment, reminding you to embrace the now, or just being there to listen unconditionally to you. **There is no shame in asking for help, on the contrary – it is a sign of strength.**

Realize that everyone has problems, even the people that seem the most together to you. It is often said that if everyone put their troubles in a bag and then drew out new ones we'd want our old troubles back.

As you open up, communicate facts about the condition, pointing the individual in the direction of online resources or books to give them a better understanding of what you are going through. Give them the 'Loved One's Guide' included at the end of this book to help them better understand just what Eyelash Trichotillomania is and what you are going through. Then give them clear instructions on how they can help you. Explain that empty words such as 'just stop' are actually very frustrating and do more harm than good. Give the person a good idea of exactly what actions you need from them and in what situations.

Having a 'buddy' to help you can be a powerful tool to fight the loneliness and help you when things get tough.

Facts About Hair Growth

Human hair naturally falls out and therefore your hair WILL grow back, even after being repeatedly pulled out. Here are some facts to about hair growth:

○ Human hair grows approximately 1/4 to 1/2 inch per month, or 6 inches per year.

○ Heat, as well as Vitamin D from the sun can stimulate growth, so getting sun on your face will make your eyelashes grow back faster.

○ Your body is constantly shedding hair. Hair follicles go through three phases during their life cycle: the anagen phase for about three years, a transitional phase and the telogen phase for about three months, when hair rests. Once this phase ends, the hair is shed.

○ Eyelashes naturally grow, fall out, and grow back again. Eyelashes also go through the 3 phases of hair: growth, transition, and resting phases. The 1st phase is when eyelashes grow and lasts up to a maximum of 45 days. After which, they go through the 2nd phase which may last up to 3 weeks, when the eyelashes stop growing. In the 3rd phase, the lashes are not growing and stay for approximately 100 days before they then fall out.

o It normally takes up to 8 weeks for an eyelash to

grow back fully.

Recommended Resources

I cannot emphasize enough how much reading can help you in your Eyelash Trichotillomania treatment. Not only should you read to be more informed about your condition and the various possibilities for treatment, but also as inspiration and to help guide you to find a more positive and happy life. Using other people's energy to boost you up is a great way of getting out of the blues or building the positive outlook that is so essential in treating eyelash pulling.

The more informed you are and the more contact with others the better your chances are of beating your condition. It's important to know that you are not alone and the anonymous contact with others can help with the feelings of loneliness and isolation that can individuals suffering from Eyelash Trichotillomania may experience from time to time.

Use the following as additional resources in your treatment.

1. Books

The Power of Habit - Charles Duhigg

Fascinating research about 'habits' (and while we know that eyelash pulling is not a 'habit' as such, he does go into repetitive behaviors).

The Success Principles – Jack Canfield

This is a more general work about success in life, however the principles are great and it has a wonderful upbeat message that leaves you with a positive message for the future.

Stop Me Because I Can't Stop Myself – Jon Grant

An informative book on impulse control disorders, Dr. Grant's research is funded by the National Institute of Mental Health.

Pretty Little Things – Cheryl Strayed

Funny, insightful and compassionate. This book will show you that we all have our issues and give you strength to keep working towards a better life. "A balm for everything life throws our way."

2. Websites

http://www.trich.org

Full of information, seminars and contacting others about OCDs.

http://www.ocduk.org/

Based in the UK, this charity helps individuals with obsessive-compulsive disorders.

Notes

Using the Trich Stop System Worksheet and Journal

Use the following steps along with the Trich Stop Manual and Trich Stop Oil to put a structure and plan in place to beat your condition. While we have included several pages that you can fill in so that you can get started right away, we recommend that you make some photocopies of the workbook for continued use.

1. Recognize The Condition

Acknowledge that you have a problem. The first thing to realize is that you suffer from treatable disorder, not something due to willpower or lack thereof. The disorder arises as a result of genetic makeup, moods, and your background and is a condition in need of treating, not something to beat yourself up over.

2. Identify When You Pull

Know your triggers. When do you pull your eyelashes out? In the evening when watching tv or reading? When speaking to your ex-husband on the phone? When working on your thesis? Make a list of your triggers and next to each write down an alternative activity that would make you feel better in these contexts.

3. Write Down When You Pull and Keep a Journal

Keep a journal or a chart of your eyelash and eyebrow pulling episodes. Through writing you can get a good idea of the times, the triggers, and the impact of your eyelash pulling. This is a good way of relieving yourself of the guilt and shame, and of expressing how the eyelash pulling is impacting your life in general. You will begin to identify your weak moments and mental states. By being more aware of these moments and feelings you will begin to master them. You will also want to use a journal to express your emotions.

Write out a list of the consequences you've experienced as a result of the eyelash pulling.

4. Structure Your Treatment

Don't leave your daily activities to chance. Having a defined daily schedule to follow will give you the support you need and help you focus on your actions. Follow your daily schedule as closely as possible to help you in developing new habits. However allow yourself the flexibility to change your schedule if you find that it doesn't work for you until you hit a rhythm that best suits your lifestyle.

If you have to break your rhythm one day because of extenuating circumstances (travel, your family needs you, etc), then don't get too hung about it, but make sure you get back into the swing of things as soon as you can.

Write down your daily schedule and put it in a place that you can refer to it easily (the refrigerator door for example).

Some examples:

Morning – wake and have a few minutes in bed visualizing a successful, happy non-pulling day. Apply some natural conditioning essential oils or Trich Stop Oil before getting dressed. Write in your journal for 2 pages, without stopping. Don't worry about what you have written, just use it as a way of emptying your mind. Take 10 minutes before your day begins to meditate and prepare for the day.

Afternoon – set aside some time to write in your journal and fill out your workbook. Go for a walk, exercise or work on your hobby.

Evening – red flag as this is a risk time, so be aware of when triggers might happen, such as watching tv or reading. Have your oil ready to rub in and be aware. Prepare an activity that you can do if you find yourself in a weak moment. Use this down time to read some inspirational books on your condition, but also on a happy life and philosophy in general. Give yourself a mini sauna using essential oils and natural plants.

Night – reflect on the positive parts of your day and the things that went well. Any negative thoughts should be acknowledged, reduced and eliminated from your mind as they enter.

Now create your own using the pages in the workbook.

5. How to fill out the worksheet and journal

Keep a regular journal, filling it out daily with your eyelash pulling related experiences. We have included the first few pages to get you started.

Comments and observations from others:

Include comments you have endured and any observations friends, family or strangers have made about your appearance or condition, and how you felt.

Behavioral consequences to my pulling

Include any behavior that is a consequence of your condition (having to go to great lengths with eyeliner, having difficulty in finding the right shade of eyebrow pencil, etc.), and how you felt.

Relationship consequences to my pulling

Include the relationship consequences, such as not going on a date or to spending time with people because you're afraid they will find out about your eyelash pulling, and how you felt.

Triggers

Make a list of your triggers and next to each write down an alternative activity that would make you feel better in these contexts.

Tracking Chart

Fill out a chart like the one on the next page to track your

pulling behavior and emotions:

Date, time	Place	Trigger	How many hairs pulled	What was used to pull?	Thoughts	Feelings	Possible other activities

My Trich Stop Success Journal

My Top Tips for Getting Control

1. Recognize the condition, read up, do some research, really understand what you are confronting

2. Believe that it is possible to get your condition under control. Surround yourself with a positive support group and have faith.

3. Get a systematized plan in place. You can't just expect to stop, and surely we all know that 'willpower' is just not the answer. So you need to put a very clear plan in place.

4. Try different methods to see which one works for you. Every person is different, so methods will have differing results depending on the person. Try visualization, journalizing, and mediation. All of these methods have their merits. The best option in my opinion is to have a mix of methods.

5. Use something (natural) to stroke on the area. For me this was key because it helped me not only relieve the nagging feelings, but more importantly, it helped me rewire my brain and change the pulling action to a stroking action. I still find myself stroking or rubbing when I can feel an urge coming on. That is a heck of a lot better than pulling!

6. Cut out chemicals in your diet (processed foods, sugars, etc) and in your cosmetics. And get as healthy as you can.

7. Finally, be KIND TO YOUR SELF. We all know that getting these conditions under control is very difficult. So if you slip up, then give yourself a break, pick yourself up, dust yourself off and start again. Stopping is a gradual process, so be happy with any progress you have made and keep at it. Don't get discouraged.

My Personal Daily Schedule

Morning: -

_____

_____

_____

_____

_____

_____

_____

_____

Afternoon: -

_____

_____

_____

_____

_____

_____

_____

_____

_____

Evening:

_____

_____

_____

_____

_____

_____

_____

_____

My Personal Stress Reducing Activities

_____

_____

_____

_____

_____

_____

_____

_____

_____

_____

_____

_____

_____

Comments and observations from others

Comments:

_____

_____

_____

My feelings:

_____

_____

_____

Comments:

_____

_____

_____

My feelings:

_____

_____

_____

Comments:

_____

_____

_____

My feelings:

_____

_____

_____

Comments:

_____

_____

_____

My feelings:

_____

_____

_____

Comments:

_____

_____

_____

My feelings:

_____

_____

_____

Comments:

_____

_____

_____

My feelings:

_____

_____

_____

Behavioral consequences to my pulling

Behavior:

_____

_____

_____

My feelings:

_____

_____

_____

Behavior:

_____

_____

_____

My feelings:

_____

_____

_____

Behavior:

_____

_____

_____

My feelings:

_____

_____

_____

Behavior:

_____

_____

_____

My feelings:

_____

_____

_____

Behavior:

_____

_____

_____

My feelings:

_____

_____

Behavior:

_____

_____

_____

My feelings:

_____

_____

_____

Relationship consequences to my pulling

Behavior:

_____

_____

_____

My feelings:

_____

_____

_____

Behavior:

_____

_____

_____

My feelings:

_____

_____

_____

Behavior:

_____

_____

_____

My feelings:

_____

_____

_____

Behavior:

_____

_____

_____

My feelings:

_____

_____

_____

Behavior:

_____

_____

_____

My feelings:

_____

_____

_____

Behavior:

_____

_____

_____

My feelings:

_____

_____

_____

Triggers

Trigger:

_____

_____

_____

Alternative activity:

_____

_____

_____

Trigger:

_____

_____

_____

Alternative activity:

_____

_____

_____

Trigger:

_____

_____

_____

Alternative activity:

_____

_____

_____

Trigger:

_____

_____

_____

Alternative activity:

_____

_____

_____

Trigger:

_____

_____

_____

Alternative activity:

_____

_____

_____

Trigger:

_____

_____

_____

Alternative activity:

_____

_____

_____

Tracking Chart

Date, time	Place	Trigger	How many hairs pulled	What used was to pull?	Thoughts	Feelings	Possible other activities

Date, time	Place	Trigger	How many hairs pulled	What used was to pull?	Thoughts	Feelings	Possible other activities

Notes

Notes

If you liked this...

We hope you have found this book helpful. If you would like to know more about how you can continue to fight against Eyelash Trichotillomania, then contact us at info@foxwellassociates.com.

A Special Offer

As one of our Trich Stop community we'd like to extend to you these special offers:

- a 10% discount on the Trich Stop Oil. Trich Stop Oil is an all natural oil made from ingredients such as olive oil, French lavender, jojoba, citrus, basil, rosemary and other essential oils and plant essences. It is used to soothe follicles, reduce urges, promote eyelash and eyebrow growth and most importantly, encourage behavior modification, helping you to change your pulling habit to caressing.

- a 10% discount on the Trich Stop Amino Acid Supplement. Amino Acids are increasingly seen as a powerful part of Trichotillomania treatment. Our NAC Supplement has been developed with a highly reputable supplier with obsessive-compulsive disorders in mind.

If you are interested in either (or both) of these offers, simply use the code 'BEATTRICH' on the www.trichotillomaniastop.com website when prompted. Your discount will be automatically applied.

We'd Love to Hear from You

We believe that a community is a powerful thing. If you have any thoughts, comments, feedback or suggestions then please feel free to send them through to us at comments@foxwellassociates.com. If there is anything you have done that you think would be beneficial to other Trichotillomania sufferers, or unique ways you have used the ideas presented here, then send them in. Here at Trich

Stop, we are always happy to work as a team.

The Trich Stop Loved One's Guide

A Word to Family and Friends

Firstly, let me congratulate you on your pro-activeness and willingness to help your loved one through Eyelash Trichotillomania. Reading this, understanding the condition and empathizing is the first step to helping them in their battle against eyelash pulling. I also encourage you to read the rest of 'Eyelash Pulling' for more information and to better understand the different methods your loved one will be using. Whether they have been battling with Trichotillomania for many years, or has just begun to suffer from this condition, as a friend or member of the family you must take an active position today in helping your loved one beat Eyelash Trichotillomania.

I began suffering from eyelash pulling as a young child. However, my family did not recognize it at the time and nothing was done to deal with my condition, which eventually made it much more difficult for me in the long run. I suffered from my condition for over 35 years before finally finding a set of treatments that helped me become an 'ex-eyelash puller'. I can only think that if my family had been more aware, or more supportive, I would not have suffered for so long.

Your friend or relative will need your help, encouragement, patience, guidance and wisdom. But together I know that you can beat eyelash pulling. Who knows, perhaps even your relationship will benefit from working through this difficult challenge together.

All my best for you and your loved one,

Amy

Why Does My Loved One Suffer From This?

Eyelash Trichotillomania is an impulse control disorder. Sufferers are unable to stop this behavior, and the behavior is often self-destructive and distressing to the sufferer.

It is important to understand from the very beginning that Eyelash Trichotillomania is serious condition and more than just a nervous habit, which can be controlled through simply by deciding to stop.

Research of causes and treatments of Trichotillomania are still in the early stages, and no one is really sure what causes eyelash pulling. Most likely there are several different causes that may act separately or as a combined cause. It could be a neurobiological disorder and may be linked to one's genetic makeup. At times it is triggered by stress, anxiety and depression. Eyelash pullers pull because it feels good or fills some kind of need, but hardly ever because they want to become ugly or to purposely disfigure themselves.

Trichotillomania is believed to affect 2-5% of the population (you see, your loved one is not alone, or really that strange at all!) and 80-90% of reported cases are women, although in children the percentage is closer to a 50-50% ratio of girls to boys. The average age of onset is 11, however pulling can start at any age. Some people may stop on their own. However, many do not, and we encourage friends and relatives to understand the condition fully and to get involved in finding a treatment as soon as possible. The earlier neural patterns that develop during habits are altered, the easier it will be for the sufferer to be cured.

Common Feelings

As a friend or relative you will go through a variety of emotions, and just the ups and downs can be very wearing on sufferers and loved ones alike. You will feel frustration and despair, followed by elation when they start to improve, only to be disappointed when he or she starts pulling again. You will probably not understand what is going on and not really believe that the eyelash puller cannot control his or her behavior. You will most likely feel embarrassed by their appearance, sometimes to the extent of not wanting to talk about it, even with health care professionals. You will probably also experience guilt, as if there is something that you can do differently that would change the situation. You may also feel overwhelmed and confused by all of the conflicting advice and thoughts. **While all of these feelings are perfectly natural reactions, you must understand**

the condition fully in order to dispel these emotions and replace them with more constructive and positive feelings of hope, encouragement and positivism.

Belief is key in treatment of habits and obsessive-compulsive conditions. There have been many studies around why groups such as Alcoholics Anonymous are effective, and there is very strong evidence that an important factor is seeing others who have achieved a goal. **Being in a group that cultivates positivism and a 'can do' attitude has a huge impact on eventual success.** Therefore it is important to both stay positive for your friend or relative, as well as to surround them with positive support groups and role models.

Just remember, the sufferer will also be going through his or her own set of (often very similar) emotions, such as shame, guilt and not being able to understand why he or she cannot stop.

In this case you need to be a strong support for your loved one to be able to work through their emotions with you, without judgment or your own baggage interfering. In order to do this you must understand the condition and have complete compassion for the sufferer. Have you ever tried to stop smoking, chew on your fingernails or follow a diet? If so, then you know that often these things are much more difficult than they look. With this in mind, put yourself in the sufferer's shoes and exhibit compassion at all times when dealing with them.

Compassion is key.

Your friend or family member will pick up on your own attitude and outlook. A sense of confidence and belief in them, coupled with compassion and understanding will make recovery not only possible, but a less stressful and isolating time for all concerned.

Your attitude and outlook means everything, and your friend or loved one will follow your lead.

Helping your Loved One

No matter what the age of the sufferer, or your relationship to them, your approach should be similar. Your goal is to establish trust in each other, to show your confidence in them and to boost their self-esteem when they are feeling low.

Explaining what Eyelash Trichotillomania is, how many people of all sorts are affected, sharing the websites, resources and stories of others and thus showing him that he is not a freak is an important first step. Or perhaps he or she has already done the work and merely wants to show you the amount of people and resources that exist for hair pullers. **Listen openly and actively.**

Explaining to your friend or family member that you understand what they are going through and that you know that they can't 'just stop' will be a relief to the eyelash puller who surely feels that no one understands him. You will become a safe haven for your loved one who will come to you more and more often for help. Show them that you are there to help them put a structured plan in place and that this will be a gradual, but positive process. Often verbalizing your own experience of difficulties in changing your behavior (whether it be dieting, nail biting, smoking, etc) can show your friend or family member better than through words that you understand his situation and that he truly is not alone.

Do not set time limits or ultimatums, or use rewards. These will only put pressure on the sufferer and often result in more lost confidence when they cannot reach the goals that have been set.

Above all, never chastise, ridicule or punish anyone in hopes that you can control their condition. This will not work and will only backfire, making them more secretive and more ashamed, exacerbating the problem.

All of your actions should be based on building confidence and trust. When in doubt, ask yourself if the message you are sending is a constructive, collaborative and positive one that will set your loved on up for success.

Your Philosophy as a Friend or Relative

This is a good time to reevaluate your philosophy as a friend or family member. Do you even have one? To be a good friend or relative, it is important to have a well thought out philosophy of how you want your relationship to be; a philosophy that is in line with your beliefs and goals. A philosophy will give very important coherence to your relationships, but will also help you in those frustrating moments when you aren't sure how to react. In these moments you can always fall back on your beliefs and ask yourself what actions would be in line with that philosophy. In my relationships, I have found that the philosophy that I established at the very beginning of my adulthood, a philosophy of kindness, respect and loyalty has helped me throughout all of my relationships.

Your philosophy as a friend and family member and how you treat others around other subjects will have an impact on your ability to deal with your loved one's eyelash pulling condition. A good way to develop your philosophy is to read books (see our list of recommended resources), consult blogs, talk to others that you admire, discuss with your relationship goals with others, and observe how others create constructive relationships.

Think about what values you want to instill in your relationships and how to exhibit these to others (people treat us as we expect to be treated), what kind of relationship you see with them in the long run, etc.

For eyelash pulling treatments, having a philosophy of caring support, encouraging confidence and belief, and establishing a strong structure for your friend or relative to function in are the most effective things you can do.

Treatment and support

Just as there are many different sufferers of Eyelash Trichotillomania, there are many different types of treatments, from medication to self-awareness training. There is no known 'cure' for eyelash pulling but there are treatment options available. Discovering ways to control eyelash pulling impulses can help a patient become pull free. Cognitive behavior therapy, stress-control medications, and hair pulling support groups have all proven as an effective way to control symptoms. Cognitive Behavior Therapy trains patients in self-monitoring, identifying and responding to high-risk solutions, assessing the function of the pull, confronting realizations, and developing mindfulness.

I suggest working with a mix of methods in order to find the one or combination that is most effective for your friend of family member's particular case. Often a combination of treatments will prove to be the most effective.

Most importantly, it is important for those who suffer from Trichotillomania to know that although it can be difficult to stop eyelash pulling, it is possible!

Therapy or no?

While we encourage suffers to give therapy a go (after all, we use accountants and lawyers for specialized help, why not a therapist), many individuals (and relatives or friends for that matter) balk at therapy. It seems to concretize the abnormality and shame. We suggest starting with a home program to give the sufferer some confidence and structure in the privacy of their own home. Once they are feeling good with the advances they are making, you can try a therapist and see if this is right for the sufferer. **Above all do not force a friend or relative to see a therapist or do anything in their treatment that they do not want to do.**

A sufferer's acceptance is often gradual, and respecting their own rhythm sends the important message that you have confidence in them.

Setbacks and how to deal with them

One last word on setbacks: setbacks are a normal part of the process and you should be prepared, and prepare your loved one for them. Aim for gradual healing rather than a radical cold turkey approach, which will only cause frustration and loss of confidence. **Retraining the neural patterns as well as putting healing systems in place takes time, so allow your family and friends the time to heal together.** When your loved one has a setback, don't make a big deal out of it. Just pick yourselves back up, dust yourselves off, explain the gradual nature of recovery and start again. Explain that having been able to make any progress at all shows that it is possible. Now it just needs to become ingrained behavior, which it will, with enough time and practice.

Most of all teach your loved one to be kind to himself.

Trich Stop Tips

Reduce stress

Keep the household and environment as stress free as possible. While this is easier said than done, make an effort to keep the atmosphere a low-key as possible.

Keep changes to a minimum

Try to keep to an established rhythm.

Turn off the TV

TV allows for negative messaging, trance-like states and inactivity. Encourage the individual to do something constructive instead.

Consider getting your loved one a pet

Pets are great for reducing stress, increasing activity and giving unconditional love.

Remove mirrors

Removing any possible mirrors will help the individual stop focusing on their appearance.

Remember

- Show your confidence in the individual

- Compassion and belief are ESSENTIAL

- Encourage the sufferer to try many different methods to find the ones that work best for him or her

- NEVER tell the individual that they can 'Just Stop' if they really wanted to

- Listen actively

- Never chastise, punish, ridicule or force the sufferer in any way

- Reduce stress in the household

- Eliminate change and keep things as constant as possible, helping the sufferer to put a treatment structure in place

- Encourage hobbies, exercise or other activities

- o Encourage the individual to modify his pulling behavior to stroking (using some sort of all natural oil) on order to develop new neural pathways and instill long lasting results

How to Help with Treatments

Follow your loved one's lead when helping them work through their condition.

Firstly, encourage them to use a journal as they would like – writing in it, doodling, whatever helps them express themselves. Don't ask to see their journal or any private writings and don't look at them unless they ask you to. Don't even 'check up' to see if they have been writing in their journal. This is a moment to establish trust and confidence, which will, in turn, help them discover confidence in themselves.

Also help them embrace this aspect of their unique personality and life. Explain that this is part of who they are, and that there is nothing wrong with it. That Eyelash

Trichotillomania is a legitimate condition that they should not be ashamed of. Encourage them to accept, and then let go.

Suggest they keep some kind of oil (we recommend the Trich Stop Oil – see the end of this book for a special offer) to discreetly use then they are having urges. It is important to help them begin the reflex of stroking rather than pulling.

Remember - this is their journey and you are there only as support.

Recommended Resources

I cannot emphasize enough how much reading can help you understand Trichotillomania and your loved one's condition. Read to be informed, but also as inspiration to help you through this difficult situation.

Use the following as additional resources.

1. Books

A Good Enough Parent - Bruno Bettleheim

An encouraging and uplifting look at parenthood, this book will give you a guilt free philosophy to be the best parent you can be.

The Power of Habit - Charles Duhigg

Fascinating research about 'habits' (and while we know that hair pulling is not a 'habit' as such, he does go into repetitive behaviors).

The Success Principles – Jack Canfield

This is a more general work about success in life, however the principles are great and it has a wonderful upbeat message that leaves you with a positive message for the future to pass on to your loved one.

Stop Me Because I Can't Stop Myself – Jon Grant

An informative book on impulse control disorders. Dr. Grant's research is funded by the National Institute of Mental Health.

2. Websites

http://www.trich.org

A site full of information and resources about OCDs.

http://www.ocduk.org/

Based in the UK, this charity helps individuals with obsessive-compulsive disorders.

3. Trich Stop

You are also welcome to contact us directly at

info@foxwellassociates.com for any further information.

Notes

17899497R00111

Printed in Great Britain
by Amazon